How to End Infections Completely Using Amoxicillin Antibiotic Pills

by:

Dr. Jackie L. Mauldin

Contents

Chapter 1

Understanding Infections and Antibiotics

1.1 What Are Infections?

Infections are a broad category of medical conditions caused by the invasion and multiplication of harmful microorganisms in the body. These microorganisms, known as pathogens, can include bacteria, viruses, fungi, and parasites. When they enter the body, they can disrupt normal bodily functions, leading to a variety of symptoms and health issues.

Infections can occur in different parts of the body and can vary in severity. Some common examples of infections include:

1. Bacterial Infections: These are caused by bacteria and can affect various organs and systems in the body. Examples include strep throat, urinary tract infections (UTIs), and bacterial pneumonia.
2. Viral Infections: These are caused by viruses and can range from common colds and influenza (flu) to more serious conditions like HIV, hepatitis, and COVID-19.

3. Fungal Infections: These are caused by fungi and can affect the skin, nails, mouth (oral thrush), and other parts of the body. Examples include athlete's foot and vaginal yeast infections.
4. Parasitic Infections: These are caused by parasites and can be transmitted through contaminated food, water, or insect bites. Examples include malaria, giardiasis, and trichomoniasis.

Infections can be transmitted from person to person through various means, such as direct contact with infected individuals, airborne droplets, contaminated food or water, or insect bites. Some infections can also be acquired from the environment or through contact with animals.

The body's immune system plays a crucial role in defending against infections. It recognizes and fights off the invading pathogens to prevent the infection from spreading and causing further harm. In some cases, the immune system may successfully eliminate the infection without the need for medical intervention. However, in more severe or persistent infections, medical treatment may be necessary, often involving the use of antibiotics, antiviral drugs, antifungal medications, or other specific therapies.

Proper hygiene, vaccination, and following medical guidelines for preventing and managing infections are essential in reducing the risk of getting sick and maintaining overall health. If you suspect you have an infection or experience symptoms such as fever, pain, swelling, or unusual discharge, it is crucial to seek medical attention promptly to receive appropriate diagnosis and treatment.

1.2 Types of Infections

Infections can be categorized based on the type of pathogens that cause them. The main types of infections are:

1. Bacterial Infections:

Bacterial infections are caused by various types of bacteria. These microorganisms can invade different parts of the body and cause a wide range of illnesses, from mild to severe. Common bacterial infections include:

- Strep throat
- Urinary tract infections (UTIs)
- Bacterial pneumonia
- Skin infections (e.g., cellulitis)
- Bacterial gastroenteritis (food poisoning)
- Tuberculosis (TB)

2. Viral Infections:

Viral infections are caused by viruses, which are smaller than bacteria and need a host cell to replicate. They can lead to a variety of illnesses, from common colds to serious conditions. Some common viral infections include:

- Influenza (flu)
- Common cold
- COVID-19 (coronavirus disease)
- HIV/AIDS
- Hepatitis (e.g., hepatitis A, B, C)
- Herpes (e.g., cold sores, genital herpes)

3. Fungal Infections:

Fungal infections are caused by fungi, which are organisms that can thrive in moist environments. They can affect the skin, nails, mucous membranes, and internal organs. Common fungal infections include:

- Athlete's foot (tinea pedis)
- Ringworm (tinea corporis)
- Vaginal yeast infections (candidiasis)
- Oral thrush (oral candidiasis)
- Fungal nail infections (onychomycosis)

4. Parasitic Infections:

Parasitic infections are caused by parasites, which are organisms that live on or inside a host organism and obtain nutrients from it. They can be transmitted through contaminated food, water, insect bites, or direct contact. Some common parasitic infections include:

- Malaria
- Giardiasis
- Trichomoniasis
- Toxoplasmosis
- Intestinal worms (e.g., roundworm, hookworm)

5. Prion Diseases:

Prion diseases are caused by abnormal, misfolded proteins called prions. These proteins can induce other proteins in the brain to fold abnormally, leading to neurodegenerative disorders. Examples include:

- Creutzfeldt-Jakob disease (CJD)
- Variant Creutzfeldt-Jakob disease (vCJD)
- Bovine spongiform encephalopathy (mad cow disease)

Each type of infection can present with specific symptoms and require different approaches for diagnosis and treatment. Proper management, prevention, and timely medical intervention are crucial in controlling the spread and impact of infections. Vaccination, good hygiene practices, and responsible antibiotic use are some of the preventive measures that can help reduce the incidence of infections.

1.3 Introduction to Antibiotics

Antibiotics are a class of powerful medications used to treat bacterial infections and some specific fungal infections. They have revolutionized modern medicine and saved countless lives since their discovery in the early 20th century. The word "antibiotic" comes from the Greek words "anti," meaning "against," and "bios," meaning "life."

The discovery of the first antibiotic, penicillin, by Sir Alexander Fleming in 1928, marked a significant milestone in medical history. Penicillin was derived from the Penicillium mold and proved to be highly effective in treating bacterial infections, particularly those caused by the bacteria Staphylococcus and Streptococcus.

How Antibiotics Work:

Antibiotics work by targeting specific components or processes within bacteria, disrupting their growth and reproduction, ultimately leading to their destruction. Different antibiotics have different mechanisms of action, but some common ways in which antibiotics work include:

1. Inhibition of Cell Wall Formation: Many antibiotics, such as penicillin and cephalosporins, target the synthesis of bacterial cell walls. Bacterial cells need a strong and intact cell wall to maintain their structure and protect them from bursting. By disrupting cell wall formation, antibiotics cause the bacteria to weaken and eventually die.
2. Inhibition of Protein Synthesis: Other antibiotics, like tetracyclines and macrolides, interfere with the production of bacterial proteins essential for their survival and reproduction. Without these proteins, the bacteria cannot function properly and eventually perish.
3. Inhibition of DNA/RNA Synthesis: Some antibiotics, such as fluoroquinolones, target bacterial DNA or RNA synthesis. By blocking these processes, the bacteria are unable to replicate and cannot spread further.

It's important to note that antibiotics are not effective against viral infections, such as the common cold, flu, or most cases of COVID-19. Viruses are different from bacteria, and their structure and life cycle are distinct. Antiviral medications specifically target viral infections.

Responsible Use of Antibiotics:

While antibiotics are highly effective in treating bacterial infections, their misuse and overuse can lead to the development of antibiotic resistance. Antibiotic resistance occurs when bacteria evolve and become resistant to the effects of antibiotics, making infections harder to treat. To combat this growing global health threat, it is essential to use antibiotics responsibly. This includes:

- Taking antibiotics only when prescribed by a healthcare professional.
- Completing the full course of antibiotics as prescribed, even if symptoms improve.
- Avoiding the sharing of antibiotics with others.
- Not using antibiotics to treat viral infections.

The Future of Antibiotics:

Antibiotic resistance is a significant concern, and the development of new antibiotics has slowed in recent years. Researchers and pharmaceutical companies are actively working to discover new antibiotics and alternative therapies to combat resistant bacteria. In addition to developing new drugs, promoting infection prevention strategies and adopting prudent antibiotic prescribing practices are essential to safeguarding the efficacy of existing antibiotics for future generations.

1.4 Role of Amoxicillin in Treating Infections

Amoxicillin is a widely used and effective antibiotic belonging to the penicillin class. It plays a crucial role in treating various bacterial infections, and its versatility makes it one of the most commonly prescribed antibiotics worldwide. The primary role of amoxicillin in treating infections stems from its ability to target and inhibit the growth of certain bacteria.

1. Bacterial Infections: Amoxicillin is primarily prescribed for the treatment of bacterial infections caused by susceptible organisms. It is effective against a wide range of bacteria, including Streptococcus, Staphylococcus, Haemophilus influenzae, Escherichia coli (E. coli), and some strains of Salmonella and Shigella.

2. Respiratory Infections: Amoxicillin is frequently used to treat respiratory infections such as:
   - Sinusitis: Inflammation of the sinuses.
   - Tonsillitis: Infection and inflammation of the tonsils.
   - Bronchitis: Infection of the airways (bronchi).
   - Pneumonia: Infection of the lungs.

3. Ear Infections: Amoxicillin is commonly prescribed for bacterial ear infections (otitis

media), which can affect both children and adults.

4. Urinary Tract Infections (UTIs): Amoxicillin can be effective in treating uncomplicated urinary tract infections caused by susceptible bacteria.

5. Skin and Soft Tissue Infections: It is also used to treat various skin and soft tissue infections, including cellulitis.

6. Dental Infections: Amoxicillin is often prescribed for dental infections, including abscesses and dental caries.

Mechanism of Action: Like other penicillin antibiotics, amoxicillin works by interfering with the bacterial cell wall synthesis. It inhibits the transpeptidase enzyme, which is responsible for cross-linking the peptidoglycan chains in the bacterial cell wall. As a result, the bacterial cell wall becomes weak and unable to withstand the internal pressure, leading to cell lysis and death of the bacteria.

Amoxicillin is available in various forms, including oral capsules, tablets, chewable tablets, and liquid suspension, making it convenient for different age groups and patients with swallowing difficulties.

It's essential to note that amoxicillin is not effective against viral infections, such as the common cold or the flu. It should only be used when prescribed by a healthcare professional to treat bacterial infections. Additionally, as with all antibiotics, responsible use of amoxicillin is crucial to prevent the development of antibiotic resistance.

Chapter 2

The Mechanism of Amoxicillin

2.1 How Amoxicillin Works in the Body

Amoxicillin is a broad-spectrum antibiotic that belongs to the penicillin class. It works by interfering with the growth and replication of bacteria, ultimately leading to their destruction. The mechanism of action of amoxicillin involves targeting the bacterial cell wall, a vital structure that provides strength and rigidity to the bacteria.

1. Bacterial Cell Wall: Many bacteria have a cell wall surrounding their cell membrane, which plays a crucial role in maintaining the structural integrity of the bacteria. The cell wall is primarily composed of a complex molecule called peptidoglycan.

2. Inhibition of Cell Wall Synthesis: Amoxicillin exerts its antibacterial effects by inhibiting the synthesis of peptidoglycan, a critical component of the bacterial cell wall. Specifically, amoxicillin interferes with an enzyme called transpeptidase or penicillin-binding protein (PBP). This enzyme is responsible for cross-linking the peptidoglycan chains, providing the bacterial cell wall with its strength and stability.

3. Weakening the Cell Wall: In the presence of amoxicillin, the transpeptidase enzyme is unable to carry out its usual function of cross-linking the peptidoglycan strands. As a result, the newly formed bacterial cell wall becomes structurally weak and cannot withstand the internal pressure exerted by the bacterial cytoplasm.
4. Cell Lysis and Bacterial Death: With a weakened cell wall, the bacteria become susceptible to osmotic pressure, causing the cell to take up excess water. The increased pressure within the bacterial cell leads to cell lysis, where the cell membrane ruptures, and the contents of the bacteria leak out. This process ultimately results in the death of the bacteria.

It's important to note that amoxicillin is effective against a wide range of Gram-positive and some Gram-negative bacteria, but it is not effective against all types of bacteria. Additionally, amoxicillin's activity is limited to actively growing bacteria, as it targets cell wall synthesis during bacterial replication.

Responsible Use of Amoxicillin:

To ensure the efficacy of amoxicillin and minimize the development of antibiotic resistance, it is crucial to use the antibiotic responsibly. This includes:

1. Taking Amoxicillin as Prescribed: Always follow the dosage and administration instructions provided by your healthcare professional. Take the full course of treatment, even if you start feeling better, to ensure complete eradication of the bacterial infection.
2. Proper Diagnosis: Amoxicillin should only be used to treat bacterial infections diagnosed by a healthcare professional. It is not effective against viral infections, such as the common cold or flu.
3. Avoiding Overuse: Avoid using amoxicillin or any antibiotic unnecessarily or for conditions not requiring antibiotic treatment. Overuse of antibiotics can lead to the development of antibiotic-resistant bacteria.
4. Finishing Prescriptions: If you have leftover amoxicillin from a previous prescription, do not use it for a new infection or share it with others. Always consult your healthcare provider for a new prescription tailored to the specific infection.

By using amoxicillin responsibly and as prescribed, we can maximize its effectiveness in treating bacterial infections and contribute to the global effort to combat antibiotic resistance.

2.2 Understanding Bacterial Cell Wall Disruption

Bacterial cell wall disruption is a critical mechanism through which certain antibiotics, like amoxicillin, exert their antibacterial effects. The bacterial cell wall is a rigid and protective structure that surrounds the bacterial cell membrane, providing support and shape to the cell. It plays a crucial role in maintaining the integrity of the bacterial cell and protecting it from osmotic pressure changes.

The main component of the bacterial cell wall is a complex molecule called peptidoglycan, also known as murein. Peptidoglycan is a mesh-like structure made up of long sugar chains called glycan strands, cross-linked together by short peptide chains. This network of glycan and peptide chains forms a sturdy and strong cell wall.

Bacterial cell wall disruption occurs when antibiotics like amoxicillin interfere with the synthesis of peptidoglycan or disrupt its cross-linking, weakening the cell wall and compromising the bacterial cell's integrity. This disruption can occur through the following processes:

1. Inhibition of Transpeptidase: Amoxicillin is a β-lactam antibiotic, and it works by inhibiting an enzyme called transpeptidase or penicillin-binding protein (PBP). Transpeptidase is essential for the final stages of peptidoglycan synthesis, where it

helps cross-link the peptide chains to strengthen the cell wall. When amoxicillin binds to transpeptidase, the enzyme loses its activity, preventing proper cross-linking of peptidoglycan.

2. Weakening the Cell Wall: Without proper cross-linking of peptidoglycan, the newly formed cell wall becomes structurally weak and unable to withstand internal osmotic pressure. As a result, the bacterial cell wall becomes more susceptible to stress, including pressure changes during bacterial growth and division.

3. Activation of Autolytic Enzymes: Some antibiotics, including β-lactam antibiotics like amoxicillin, can induce the release and activation of autolytic enzymes within the bacterial cell. These enzymes further degrade the cell wall, leading to its weakening and eventual lysis of the bacterial cell.

4. Osmotic Pressure Changes: The weakened cell wall allows excess water to enter the bacterial cell, leading to an increase in osmotic pressure inside the cell. The elevated pressure causes the bacterial cell to swell and eventually burst, a process known as cell lysis.

By disrupting the bacterial cell wall, antibiotics like amoxicillin cause the bacterium to lose its structural integrity, leading to cell lysis and bacterial death. This process is selective to bacterial cells because human cells do not have peptidoglycan cell walls. As a result, amoxicillin specifically targets bacteria, making it an effective and safe antibiotic for treating bacterial infections.

2.3 Spectrum of Activity of Amoxicillin

The spectrum of activity of amoxicillin refers to the range of bacteria that the antibiotic can effectively target and treat. Amoxicillin is considered a broad-spectrum antibiotic, meaning it is effective against a wide variety of bacteria. It belongs to the penicillin class of antibiotics and is a derivative of ampicillin with enhanced antimicrobial activity.

Amoxicillin is particularly effective against Gram-positive bacteria and some Gram-negative bacteria. The term "Gram" refers to a staining technique used in microbiology to categorize bacteria based on their cell wall structure.

The spectrum of activity of amoxicillin includes the following types of bacteria:

1. Gram-Positive Bacteria: Amoxicillin is highly effective against various Gram-positive bacteria, including:

- Streptococcus species: This includes Streptococcus pyogenes (Group A streptococcus) responsible for strep throat, and Streptococcus pneumoniae, a common cause of pneumonia and ear infections.
- Staphylococcus species: Amoxicillin targets some strains of Staphylococcus, including Staphylococcus aureus (MSSA), responsible for skin infections and other diseases.

2. Some Gram-Negative Bacteria: While amoxicillin is not as effective against Gram-negative bacteria as it is against Gram-positive bacteria, it can still target some specific strains, such as:
   - Haemophilus influenzae: A bacterium that can cause respiratory tract infections, sinusitis, and ear infections.
   - Escherichia coli (E. coli): Amoxicillin is effective against certain strains of E. coli that cause urinary tract infections and gastrointestinal infections.
3. Other Bacteria: Amoxicillin may also target certain bacteria like Helicobacter pylori, which is associated with peptic ulcers and gastritis.

It's important to note that while amoxicillin has a broad spectrum of activity, it is not effective against all types of bacteria. It is not effective against bacterial strains that produce β-lactamase, an enzyme that can break down penicillin antibiotics, rendering them ineffective. In such cases, a combination of amoxicillin with a β-lactamase inhibitor, such as clavulanic acid (found in Augmentin), may be used to overcome resistance.

Additionally, amoxicillin is not effective against viral infections, such as the common cold or the flu. It should only be used to treat bacterial infections diagnosed by a healthcare professional.

Chapter 3

Safety Precautions and Contraindications

3.1 Allergies and Hypersensitivity

Allergies and hypersensitivity are immune system responses to substances that are usually harmless to most people. When a person has an allergy or hypersensitivity, their immune system reacts to these substances, known as allergens or triggers, as if they were harmful invaders. This immune response can lead to various symptoms and health problems.

Allergy:

- An allergy is an exaggerated immune response to a specific substance, often referred to as an allergen. Common allergens include pollen, dust mites, pet dander, certain foods, insect stings, and medications (e.g., antibiotics, aspirin).
- When an allergic individual comes into contact with an allergen, their immune system produces antibodies called immunoglobulin E (IgE). These IgE antibodies bind to specialized cells called mast cells and basophils.

- Upon subsequent exposure to the same allergen, the IgE antibodies on mast cells and basophils trigger the release of chemical mediators, such as histamine, into the bloodstream.
- Histamine and other mediators cause various allergic reactions, ranging from mild symptoms like sneezing, itching, and hives to more severe reactions like anaphylaxis, a life-threatening allergic emergency.

Hypersensitivity:

Hypersensitivity is a broader term that encompasses various exaggerated immune responses beyond the classical allergy mediated by IgE antibodies. Hypersensitivity reactions are classified into four types based on their underlying immune mechanisms:

- Type I Hypersensitivity (Immediate Hypersensitivity): This type is synonymous with allergies and involves IgE-mediated reactions, as described above.
- Type II Hypersensitivity (Cytotoxic Hypersensitivity): This type involves antibodies targeting specific cells or tissues, leading to cell destruction. Examples include certain autoimmune diseases and drug-induced hemolytic anemia.

- Type III Hypersensitivity (Immune Complex-Mediated Hypersensitivity): Immune complexes formed by the binding of antigens and antibodies trigger inflammatory responses that can damage tissues. Conditions like systemic lupus erythematosus (SLE) and certain types of vasculitis are examples of type III hypersensitivity.
- Type IV Hypersensitivity (Delayed-Type Hypersensitivity): This type is characterized by a delayed immune response, typically occurring 24 to 72 hours after exposure to an antigen. Contact dermatitis and some forms of allergic reactions to certain medications fall under this category.

Managing Allergies and Hypersensitivity:

The management of allergies and hypersensitivity depends on the type and severity of the reaction. Common approaches include:

- Avoidance: Identifying and avoiding allergens or triggers whenever possible is the primary strategy to prevent allergic reactions.
- Medications: Antihistamines, decongestants, nasal corticosteroids, and epinephrine (for severe allergies and

anaphylaxis) are commonly used to manage symptoms.

- Immunotherapy: Allergy shots (subcutaneous immunotherapy) or sublingual immunotherapy can help desensitize the immune system to specific allergens over time.

If you suspect you have allergies or experience severe hypersensitivity reactions, it is essential to seek medical evaluation and guidance from an allergist or immunologist to determine the specific triggers and develop a personalized management plan.

3.2 Drug Interactions with Amoxicillin

Amoxicillin, like many other medications, can interact with other drugs or substances, potentially affecting its effectiveness or increasing the risk of side effects. It's crucial to inform your healthcare provider about all the medications, supplements, and herbal products you are taking to minimize the risk of drug interactions. Some of the notable drug interactions with amoxicillin include:

1. Probenecid: Probenecid is a medication used to treat gout and can reduce the excretion of amoxicillin from the body. When taken together, probenecid can increase the blood

levels of amoxicillin, potentially leading to a higher risk of side effects.

2. Methotrexate: Methotrexate is a medication used to treat certain autoimmune conditions and cancer. When taken with amoxicillin, it can interfere with the elimination of methotrexate from the body, leading to an increased risk of methotrexate toxicity.

3. Allopurinol: Allopurinol is used to treat gout and certain types of kidney stones. Taking amoxicillin with allopurinol can increase the risk of skin rash and allergic reactions.

4. Oral Contraceptives: Some antibiotics, including amoxicillin, may reduce the effectiveness of hormonal contraceptives (birth control pills). It is advisable to use additional contraceptive methods while taking antibiotics and for a few days after completing the course.

5. Anticoagulants (Blood Thinners): Amoxicillin may increase the effects of certain anticoagulants, such as warfarin, which can lead to an increased risk of bleeding.

6. Other Antibiotics: Concurrent use of multiple antibiotics can sometimes lead to additive or overlapping effects, increasing the risk of adverse reactions.

7. Vaccines: The use of amoxicillin may reduce the effectiveness of live vaccines. It is

advisable to consult with a healthcare provider before receiving any live vaccines while on amoxicillin therapy.

It is essential to follow your healthcare provider's instructions regarding the timing and dosage of medications to avoid potential interactions. If you are taking any other medications or supplements, always consult your healthcare provider or pharmacist before starting amoxicillin to ensure safe and effective treatment. They can help you manage potential interactions and adjust dosages if necessary.

Furthermore, inform your healthcare provider if you have any allergies or a history of hypersensitivity reactions to penicillin or other antibiotics, as this information can also impact the choice of medications and treatment plan.

3.3 Precautions for Pregnant and Breastfeeding Individuals

Pregnant and breastfeeding individuals need to take special precautions when using medications, including amoxicillin, to ensure the safety and well-being of both the mother and the baby. Before taking any medication during pregnancy or while breastfeeding, it is essential to consult with a healthcare provider to weigh the potential risks and benefits. Here are some important precautions for pregnant and breastfeeding individuals regarding amoxicillin:

Precautions During Pregnancy:

1. Consult with a Healthcare Provider: Always inform your healthcare provider if you are pregnant or planning to become pregnant before starting any medication, including amoxicillin. They can assess your specific medical condition and determine if amoxicillin is safe for you and the developing baby.
2. Use Only if Necessary: Antibiotics like amoxicillin are generally considered safe during pregnancy when needed to treat bacterial infections. However, they should be used only when necessary and prescribed by a healthcare professional.
3. Avoid Self-Medication: Pregnant individuals should never self-prescribe or take any medications, including over-the-counter drugs, without proper medical advice.
4. Consideration of Alternative Medications: In some cases, healthcare providers may consider alternative antibiotics if there are concerns about amoxicillin use during pregnancy.

5. Monitoring for Side Effects: If prescribed amoxicillin during pregnancy, monitor for any side effects or adverse reactions and report them to your healthcare provider promptly.

Precautions During Breastfeeding:

1. Consult with a Healthcare Provider: Inform your healthcare provider that you are breastfeeding before taking any medications, including amoxicillin. They can assess the potential risks and benefits and determine if amoxicillin is safe to use while breastfeeding.
2. Minimal Transfer into Breast Milk: Amoxicillin is considered safe for use during breastfeeding because only a small amount is transferred into breast milk. The levels of amoxicillin in breast milk are generally not enough to harm the nursing infant.
3. Observe the Infant for Reactions: While amoxicillin is generally safe during breastfeeding, observe your baby for any unusual reactions or signs of an allergic response, such as skin rashes or digestive disturbances.
4. Timing of Medication: Taking the medication immediately after breastfeeding can help

minimize the exposure of the baby to amoxicillin in breast milk.

5. Temporary Weaning: In certain situations, a healthcare provider may recommend temporary weaning or alternative feeding methods for the baby during the course of amoxicillin treatment. However, this decision should be made under medical supervision.

Overall, the decision to use amoxicillin during pregnancy or while breastfeeding should be made with careful consideration of the individual's health condition, the potential risks, and the benefits of treatment. Open communication with a healthcare provider is essential to ensure the best possible outcome for both the mother and the baby.

3.4 Risks of Overusing and Misusing Amoxicillin

Overusing and misusing amoxicillin, or any antibiotic, can have serious consequences for both the individual taking the medication and society as a whole. The risks of overusing and misusing amoxicillin include:

1. Antibiotic Resistance: Overusing antibiotics can lead to the development of antibiotic-resistant bacteria. Bacteria can adapt and become resistant to antibiotics when they

are exposed to these drugs repeatedly or unnecessarily. When antibiotics like amoxicillin are no longer effective against bacterial infections, it becomes challenging to treat common infections effectively, leading to higher rates of treatment failure and complications.

2. Reduced Effectiveness: Misusing amoxicillin by not completing the full course of treatment can lead to incomplete eradication of bacteria. Surviving bacteria may develop resistance and cause recurrent or chronic infections that are more difficult to treat.

3. Superinfections: Overusing antibiotics can disrupt the natural balance of bacteria in the body, allowing opportunistic pathogens to grow and cause secondary infections known as superinfections. These superinfections can be more severe and resistant to treatment.

4. Allergic Reactions: Some individuals may be allergic to amoxicillin or other penicillin antibiotics. Overusing amoxicillin increases the risk of allergic reactions, ranging from mild rashes to severe anaphylaxis, a life-threatening allergic emergency.

5. Gastrointestinal Disturbances: Overusing amoxicillin can lead to disturbances in the

gut microbiota, causing gastrointestinal issues such as diarrhea and abdominal pain.

6. Increased Healthcare Costs: Antibiotic overuse contributes to increased healthcare costs due to prolonged treatments, hospitalizations, and the need for more expensive, broad-spectrum antibiotics to combat resistant infections.

7. Impact on Public Health: The overuse and misuse of antibiotics, including amoxicillin, contribute to the global problem of antibiotic resistance, making it difficult to control infectious diseases and posing a public health threat.

To mitigate these risks and preserve the effectiveness of amoxicillin and other antibiotics, it is crucial to use these medications responsibly and judiciously. Here are some important guidelines:

1. Use Antibiotics Only When Necessary: Antibiotics should be prescribed only for bacterial infections diagnosed by a healthcare professional.

2. Complete the Full Course: Always complete the full course of antibiotics as prescribed by your healthcare provider, even if you start feeling better. Stopping the medication prematurely can lead to incomplete treatment and antibiotic resistance.

3. Do Not Share Antibiotics: Never share antibiotics with others or use leftover antibiotics from previous prescriptions. Each infection requires a specific antibiotic prescribed for the individual's condition.

4. Follow Prescribing Guidelines: Healthcare providers should follow evidence-based guidelines for antibiotic prescribing and choose the most appropriate antibiotic based on the type of infection and susceptibility data.

5. Explore Alternative Treatments: For viral infections, supportive care and symptom management are more appropriate than antibiotics.

Chapter 4

Proper Dosage and Administration
4.1 Determining the Correct Dosage

Determining the correct dosage of amoxicillin, or any medication, is a critical step to ensure safe and effective treatment. The appropriate dosage depends on several factors, including the patient's age, weight, medical condition, the severity of the infection, and the type of bacteria causing the infection. It is essential to follow the dosage prescribed by a healthcare professional and not self-prescribe or adjust the dosage without proper medical guidance. Here are some general guidelines for determining the correct dosage of amoxicillin:

1. Age and Weight: For children, the dosage of amoxicillin is usually based on their weight. Healthcare providers calculate the appropriate dose based on milligrams of amoxicillin per kilogram of body weight (mg/kg). For adults, the dosage is typically based on standard adult doses.

2. Medical Condition and Severity of Infection: The dosage of amoxicillin may vary depending on the type and severity of the bacterial infection being treated. Certain

infections, such as severe respiratory or urinary tract infections, may require higher doses or more extended treatment courses.

3. Form of Amoxicillin: Amoxicillin is available in various forms, including oral capsules, tablets, chewable tablets, and liquid suspension. Each form may have different concentrations, so it is crucial to use the correct dosage form as prescribed.

4. Renal Function: In individuals with impaired kidney function, the dosage of amoxicillin may need to be adjusted to prevent potential side effects or toxicity.

5. Combination Therapy: In some cases, amoxicillin may be prescribed in combination with a β-lactamase inhibitor, such as clavulanic acid (found in Augmentin). This combination helps overcome bacterial resistance and extends the spectrum of activity against certain pathogens.

6. Timing and Frequency: The dosing schedule of amoxicillin will depend on the specific medication prescribed. Some forms of amoxicillin are taken once or twice daily, while others may require more frequent dosing.

Always follow the instructions provided by your healthcare provider regarding the dosage and administration of amoxicillin. If you have any questions or concerns about the prescribed dosage, consult your healthcare provider or pharmacist for clarification.

It is essential to complete the full course of treatment, even if you start feeling better, to ensure complete eradication of the bacterial infection and prevent the development of antibiotic resistance. Never stop taking amoxicillin or any other antibiotic prematurely without consulting your healthcare provider. Adhering to the prescribed dosage and treatment plan will help ensure the best possible outcome and minimize the risk of complications.

4.2 Amoxicillin Pill Forms and Variations

Amoxicillin, as a widely used antibiotic, is available in various pill forms and variations to accommodate different patient needs and medical conditions. Some common amoxicillin pill forms and variations include:

1. Amoxicillin Capsules: Amoxicillin is commonly available in capsule form. Capsules are typically swallowed whole with water and come in different strengths, such as 250 mg, 500 mg, and 875 mg. The specific dosage and frequency of capsules depend on the type and severity of the infection being treated.

2. Amoxicillin Tablets: Amoxicillin is also available in tablet form. Tablets may come in various strengths, similar to capsules, and are usually taken orally with water.

3. Amoxicillin Chewable Tablets: Chewable tablets are convenient for children or individuals who have difficulty swallowing pills. They are available in various flavors and can be chewed or crushed before swallowing.

4. Amoxicillin Dispersible Tablets: Dispersible tablets are designed to dissolve in water before ingestion. They are particularly suitable for children or individuals who have difficulty swallowing solid tablets.

5. Amoxicillin Extended-Release Tablets: Extended-release tablets deliver the medication gradually over an extended period, allowing for less frequent dosing. This formulation is often used for certain types of infections requiring once-daily dosing.

6. Combination Formulations: Amoxicillin is sometimes combined with a β-lactamase inhibitor, such as clavulanic acid, to enhance its effectiveness against certain bacteria and overcome resistance. This combination is commonly known as co-amoxiclav or amoxicillin-clavulanate (e.g., Augmentin).

7. Amoxicillin Powder for Oral Suspension: For patients who cannot swallow pills or need more precise dosing for children, amoxicillin is available in the form of a powder that can be reconstituted with water to form an oral suspension. The strength of the suspension depends on the amount of water added during reconstitution.

Each pill form and variation of amoxicillin has its specific instructions for administration, dosage, and storage. It is essential to follow the healthcare provider's recommendations or the instructions provided with the medication to ensure proper use and efficacy.

As with any medication, it is crucial to take amoxicillin as prescribed by a healthcare professional. Never share or use leftover amoxicillin from previous prescriptions, as each infection requires a specific dosage and treatment course tailored to the individual's condition. If you have any questions or concerns about the appropriate pill form or dosage of amoxicillin, consult your healthcare provider or pharmacist for guidance.

4.3 Administration Guidelines

Proper administration of amoxicillin is essential to ensure its effectiveness and minimize the risk of side effects. Always follow the specific instructions provided by your healthcare provider or the information on the medication label. Here are some general guidelines for administering amoxicillin:

1. Dosage: Take the prescribed dose of amoxicillin as instructed by your healthcare provider. The dosage may vary based on factors such as the type of infection, severity, age, and weight.

2. Timing: Take amoxicillin at evenly spaced intervals to maintain a consistent level of the medication in your bloodstream. If it is a twice-daily dose, try to take it approximately 12 hours apart. If it is a once-daily dose, take it at the same time each day.

3. With or Without Food: Amoxicillin can be taken with or without food, depending on the specific instructions provided by your healthcare provider. However, some formulations may be better tolerated with food to minimize gastrointestinal side effects. If you are unsure, ask your healthcare provider or pharmacist for guidance.

4. Swallowing: Swallow capsules and tablets whole with a full glass of water. Do not chew, crush, or break them unless you are specifically using chewable or dispersible tablets.

5. Chewable Tablets: If you are using chewable tablets, chew them thoroughly before swallowing. If needed, you can wash them down with a drink of water.

6. Dispersible Tablets: For dispersible tablets, follow the instructions for dissolving the tablet in water before ingestion.

7. Oral Suspension: If you are using amoxicillin powder for oral suspension, follow the reconstitution instructions carefully. Shake the suspension well before each use. Use a measuring device provided with the medication or a syringe to ensure accurate dosing.

8. Full Course: Complete the full course of treatment, even if you start feeling better before the treatment is over. Stopping the medication prematurely can lead to incomplete eradication of the bacteria and potential resistance.

9. Avoid Alcohol: While amoxicillin itself does not interact with alcohol, it's generally advisable to avoid alcohol while on antibiotics, as alcohol can interfere with the body's ability to fight infections and may worsen certain side effects.

10. Storage: Store amoxicillin as directed on the medication label. Keep it at the appropriate

temperature, away from moisture and direct sunlight. Do not use expired medication.

If you miss a dose, take it as soon as you remember, unless it is close to the time for the next scheduled dose. In that case, skip the missed dose and resume your regular dosing schedule. Do not double the dose to make up for a missed one.

Always communicate with your healthcare provider if you have any questions or concerns about the administration of amoxicillin or if you experience any side effects or unexpected symptoms during treatment. Your healthcare provider can provide specific guidance tailored to your condition to ensure safe and effective use of the medication.

4.4 Completing the Full Course of Treatment

Completing the full course of treatment is a crucial aspect of using antibiotics, including amoxicillin, to ensure effective treatment and prevent the development of antibiotic resistance. When a healthcare provider prescribes amoxicillin for a bacterial infection, they determine the appropriate duration of treatment based on the type and severity of the infection. It is essential to take the medication for the entire prescribed period, even if you start feeling better before the treatment is over.

Here are the reasons why completing the full course of treatment is important:

1. Eradication of Bacteria: Bacterial infections are caused by specific bacteria, and antibiotics like amoxicillin are designed to target and kill these bacteria. Completing the full course of treatment ensures that enough time is given to eliminate all the bacteria causing the infection. Stopping the medication prematurely can leave some bacteria alive, leading to incomplete eradication and the potential for the infection to return.

2. Preventing Resistant Bacteria: When bacteria are exposed to antibiotics but not fully eradicated, they have a chance to develop resistance to the medication. Resistant bacteria are more challenging to treat, and if they spread to other individuals, they can create a public health problem. Completing the full course of amoxicillin reduces the likelihood of antibiotic-resistant bacteria emerging and spreading.

3. Avoiding Recurrence: Infections that are not completely treated have a higher chance of recurring. Incomplete treatment can lead to a temporary suppression of symptoms, but the underlying infection may still be present. Completing the full course helps ensure that

the infection is fully cleared, reducing the risk of recurrence.

4. Promoting Optimal Health: Infections left untreated or inadequately treated can lead to more severe health complications. Completing the full course of amoxicillin helps prevent the progression of the infection and supports optimal recovery and overall health.

5. Ensuring Safety: Amoxicillin is generally safe when used as prescribed. Completing the full course of treatment reduces the risk of potential side effects and adverse reactions associated with incomplete or inappropriate antibiotic use.

If you have concerns about the medication or experience side effects during the treatment, do not stop taking amoxicillin without consulting your healthcare provider. They can assess your condition and determine if any adjustments to the treatment plan are necessary. Responsible use of antibiotics, including completing the full course of treatment, is essential in preserving their effectiveness and combating antibiotic resistance.

Chapter 5

Managing Side Effects and Adverse

5.1 Common Side Effects of Amoxicillin

Amoxicillin is generally well-tolerated, and most people do not experience significant side effects. However, like all medications, it can cause certain adverse reactions in some individuals. Common side effects of amoxicillin may include:

1. Gastrointestinal Disturbances: The most common side effects of amoxicillin are related to the gastrointestinal system and may include:
   - Nausea
   - Diarrhea
   - Abdominal pain or discomfort
   - Vomiting
2. Allergic Reactions: Some people may be allergic to amoxicillin or other penicillin antibiotics. Allergic reactions to amoxicillin can range from mild to severe and may include:
   - Skin rash or hives
   - Itching or swelling, especially of the face, lips, tongue, or throat

- Wheezing or difficulty breathing
- Anaphylaxis (a severe and life-threatening allergic reaction)
3. Thrush (Oral Candidiasis): Amoxicillin can disrupt the natural balance of microorganisms in the mouth, leading to an overgrowth of yeast called Candida. This may cause white patches or a fungal infection in the mouth known as thrush.
4. Vaginal Yeast Infections: Amoxicillin can also disturb the normal vaginal flora, leading to an overgrowth of yeast and causing vaginal yeast infections in some women.
5. Headache: Some individuals may experience mild headaches while taking amoxicillin.

It's essential to seek immediate medical attention if you experience severe allergic reactions or any other serious side effects, such as difficulty breathing, swelling, or severe skin reactions.

Most side effects of amoxicillin are mild and resolve on their own without any specific treatment. If you are experiencing bothersome side effects or have concerns about the medication, talk to your healthcare provider. They can help determine if the benefits of using amoxicillin outweigh the potential risks and may suggest alternatives if needed.

If you have a known allergy to penicillin or have experienced severe side effects from amoxicillin in the past, inform your healthcare provider before starting the medication. In such cases, your healthcare provider may choose a different antibiotic to treat your infection.

5.2 Recognizing Serious Adverse Reactions

Recognizing serious adverse reactions to medications, including amoxicillin, is essential for prompt medical attention and appropriate management. While most side effects of amoxicillin are mild and resolve on their own, some reactions can be severe and require immediate medical intervention. Here are signs of serious adverse reactions that warrant urgent medical attention:

Severe Allergic Reaction (Anaphylaxis):

- Difficulty breathing or shortness of breath
- Swelling of the face, lips, tongue, or throat
- Hives or severe skin rash
- Rapid or weak pulse
- Dizziness or lightheadedness
- Loss of consciousness

Anaphylaxis is a life-threatening allergic reaction that requires immediate emergency medical care. If you or someone else experiences any symptoms of anaphylaxis after taking amoxicillin or any other medication, call emergency services immediately.

Severe Skin Reactions:

- Severe skin rash or blistering
- Rash that spreads rapidly
- Peeling or shedding of the skin
- Fever and sore throat

Severe skin reactions can be a sign of a serious condition and may require urgent medical attention. Discontinue the use of amoxicillin and seek medical help if you develop any of these symptoms.

Severe Gastrointestinal Symptoms:

- Severe abdominal pain or cramps
- Persistent or severe diarrhea
- Bloody or black stools

While mild gastrointestinal disturbances are common with amoxicillin use, severe or persistent symptoms should be evaluated by a healthcare professional.

Liver or Kidney Problems:

- Yellowing of the skin or eyes (jaundice)
- Dark urine
- Unexplained fatigue or weakness
- Swelling in the legs, ankles, or feet

These symptoms may indicate liver or kidney problems and require medical evaluation.

Unexplained Fever:

- High or persistent fever without any other apparent cause
- Fever accompanied by other concerning symptoms

Unexplained fever while taking amoxicillin may be a sign of an underlying infection or a serious reaction and should be evaluated by a healthcare provider.

If you experience any of these serious adverse reactions while taking amoxicillin, seek immediate medical attention. Contact your healthcare provider or go to the nearest emergency room for evaluation and treatment. Prompt recognition and intervention are crucial for managing serious adverse reactions effectively. Remember to inform your healthcare provider of any known allergies or previous adverse reactions to medications before starting amoxicillin or any other antibiotic.

5.3 Strategies for Minimizing Side Effects

Minimizing side effects of amoxicillin and maximizing its effectiveness can be achieved through several strategies. Here are some tips to help reduce the risk of side effects:

1. Follow Prescribed Dosage: Take amoxicillin exactly as prescribed by your healthcare

provider. Do not alter the dosage or frequency without medical guidance. Taking the correct dosage at regular intervals helps maintain stable levels of the medication in your bloodstream, reducing the risk of side effects.

2. Take with Food: If you experience gastrointestinal discomfort while taking amoxicillin, consider taking it with food. This may help reduce stomach upset and nausea.

3. Stay Hydrated: Drink plenty of water while taking amoxicillin to stay hydrated and potentially alleviate mild side effects like nausea and diarrhea.

4. Probiotics: Consider taking probiotics or eating foods rich in probiotics, such as yogurt, during and after the course of antibiotics. Probiotics can help support the natural balance of gut bacteria and reduce the risk of antibiotic-associated diarrhea.

5. Avoid Alcohol: Avoid alcohol consumption while on antibiotics, as alcohol can interfere with the body's ability to metabolize the medication and may worsen side effects.

6. Communicate with Your Healthcare Provider: If you experience any side effects or adverse reactions while taking amoxicillin, inform your healthcare provider promptly. They can assess your symptoms and

recommend appropriate management or adjust the treatment if necessary.

7. Prevent Thrush: To reduce the risk of developing thrush (oral candidiasis), practice good oral hygiene. Rinse your mouth with water after taking amoxicillin, and consider using an antifungal mouthwash if you are prone to developing thrush.

8. Finish the Full Course: Complete the full course of amoxicillin treatment, even if you start feeling better before the treatment is over. This ensures complete eradication of the bacteria and reduces the risk of recurrence or antibiotic resistance.

9. Inform about Allergies: Inform your healthcare provider about any known allergies or previous adverse reactions to medications before starting amoxicillin or any other antibiotic. This helps them choose the most appropriate medication for your condition.

10. Monitor for Unusual Symptoms: Be vigilant for any unusual symptoms or severe reactions while taking amoxicillin. If you experience symptoms like difficulty breathing, severe rash, or swelling, seek immediate medical attention.

Remember that individual responses to medications can vary, and not everyone will experience side effects. If you have concerns or questions about amoxicillin or any other medication, discuss them with your healthcare provider. They can provide personalized advice and guidance to ensure safe and effective treatment.

Chapter 6

Lifestyle Tips for Faster Recovery

6.1 Proper Nutrition and Hydration

Proper nutrition and hydration are essential for maintaining good health and supporting the body's immune system, especially when taking medications like amoxicillin. Here are some tips for ensuring proper nutrition and hydration:

1. Eat a Balanced Diet: Consume a well-balanced diet that includes a variety of fruits, vegetables, whole grains, lean proteins, and healthy fats. A balanced diet provides essential nutrients that support overall health and help the body fight infections.

2. Include Immune-Boosting Foods: Some foods are known to boost the immune system. Incorporate foods rich in vitamin C (e.g., citrus fruits, berries, broccoli), vitamin D (e.g., fatty fish, fortified dairy products), zinc (e.g., nuts, seeds, legumes), and antioxidants (e.g., colorful fruits and vegetables) in your diet.

3. Stay Hydrated: Drink an adequate amount of water throughout the day to stay hydrated. Proper hydration helps maintain bodily

functions, supports digestion, and flushes out toxins from the body.

4. Avoid Excessive Sugar and Processed Foods: Limit the intake of sugary and processed foods, as they can weaken the immune system and contribute to inflammation.

5. Probiotics and Fermented Foods: Consider incorporating probiotics into your diet through foods like yogurt, kefir, sauerkraut, and kimchi. Probiotics support a healthy gut microbiome, which plays a vital role in immune function.

6. Avoid Alcohol and Caffeine: While moderate alcohol and caffeine consumption may be acceptable for some, excessive intake can dehydrate the body and affect overall health.

7. Meal Timing: Space out your meals and snacks throughout the day to maintain stable blood sugar levels and provide a steady source of energy.

8. Avoid Skipping Meals: Avoid skipping meals, as this can lead to nutrient deficiencies and affect your energy levels and immune function.

9. Special Considerations: If you have specific dietary needs or medical conditions, such as allergies or food intolerances, work with a

registered dietitian or healthcare provider to create a personalized nutrition plan.

10. Listen to Your Body: Pay attention to how your body responds to certain foods and adjust your diet accordingly. Everyone's nutritional needs are unique, so it's essential to listen to your body's signals.

Remember that proper nutrition and hydration are essential components of overall health and wellness. Maintaining a healthy diet and staying hydrated can complement the effectiveness of medications like amoxicillin in treating infections and support your body's natural defenses. Always consult with a healthcare provider or a registered dietitian for personalized nutrition advice and guidance, especially if you have specific health concerns or medical conditions.

6.2 Rest and Sleep

Rest and sleep are vital aspects of maintaining good health and supporting the body's ability to recover from infections and illnesses, including when taking medications like amoxicillin. Here's why rest and sleep are important:

1. Immune Function: Adequate rest and quality sleep are crucial for a well-functioning immune system. During sleep, the body

produces cytokines, which are proteins that help regulate the immune response and fight infections. Getting enough rest can enhance the body's ability to defend against infections.

2. Healing and Recovery: Rest allows the body to divert energy and resources toward healing and recovery. When you rest, the body can repair damaged tissues and rebuild its defenses, helping to recover from infections more effectively.

3. Reducing Inflammation: Chronic inflammation can hinder the body's ability to fight infections. Quality sleep can help reduce inflammation and promote a healthier immune response.

4. Energy Conservation: When the body is fighting an infection, it requires extra energy to mount an immune response. Resting conserves energy, which can be redirected towards supporting the immune system and facilitating healing.

5. Managing Stress: Adequate rest and sleep can help manage stress, as lack of sleep can increase stress levels and weaken the immune system. Stress can make the body more susceptible to infections, so managing stress through rest and relaxation is essential.

Tips for Improving Rest and Sleep:

1. Stick to a Sleep Schedule: Try to go to bed and wake up at the same time each day, even on weekends. Consistency helps regulate the body's internal clock and improves sleep quality.
2. Create a Relaxing Bedtime Routine: Establish a calming bedtime routine, such as reading, taking a warm bath, or practicing relaxation techniques like deep breathing.
3. Limit Screen Time Before Bed: Exposure to screens (phones, tablets, computers) before bedtime can disrupt sleep patterns. Aim to avoid screens for at least an hour before sleep.
4. Make Your Sleep Environment Comfortable: Ensure your sleep environment is conducive to rest, with a comfortable mattress, appropriate room temperature, and minimal light and noise.
5. Limit Caffeine and Stimulants: Avoid consuming caffeine and stimulants in the evening, as they can interfere with sleep.
6. Manage Stress: Engage in stress-reducing activities during the day, such as meditation, yoga, or spending time in nature.
7. Listen to Your Body: Pay attention to your body's signals for rest and sleep. If you feel

tired or fatigued, take breaks and get enough sleep at night.

Getting enough rest and quality sleep not only supports your body's healing processes during infections but also promotes overall well-being. If you are experiencing difficulties with sleep or suspect you have a sleep disorder, consider discussing your concerns with a healthcare provider or a sleep specialist. They can help identify potential issues and offer strategies to improve your sleep quality and overall health.

6.3 Avoiding Spread of Infections

Avoiding the spread of infections is crucial to protect yourself and others from getting sick. Whether you are currently on amoxicillin or not, here are some essential tips to prevent the spread of infections:

1. Hand Hygiene: Wash your hands frequently with soap and water for at least 20 seconds, especially after coughing, sneezing, using the restroom, or being in public places. If soap and water are not available, use hand sanitizer with at least 60% alcohol.
2. Respiratory Etiquette: Cover your mouth and nose with a tissue or your elbow when coughing or sneezing. Dispose of used

tissues properly and wash your hands immediately afterward.

3. Avoid Close Contact: Try to maintain a safe distance from people who are sick, and avoid close contact with others if you are feeling unwell.

4. Wear a Mask: Follow local health guidelines regarding the use of face masks, especially in crowded or indoor settings where physical distancing is challenging.

5. Disinfect Surfaces: Clean and disinfect frequently touched surfaces and objects regularly, including doorknobs, light switches, phones, and electronics.

6. Stay Home When Sick: If you are feeling unwell, especially if you have symptoms like fever, cough, or difficulty breathing, stay home and avoid contact with others.

7. Avoid Touching Face: Refrain from touching your eyes, nose, and mouth with unwashed hands, as this can transfer germs from surfaces to your body.

8. Practice Good Respiratory Hygiene: Encourage others to practice good respiratory hygiene, such as covering their mouth and nose when coughing or sneezing.

9. Avoid Sharing Personal Items: Avoid sharing personal items like utensils, cups, towels,

and electronic devices to prevent the spread of germs.

10. Vaccination: Stay up-to-date with vaccinations, as they can help prevent certain infections and reduce their severity if you do get sick.

11. Quarantine and Isolation: Follow public health guidelines for quarantine or isolation if you have been exposed to a contagious infection or have tested positive for one.

By following these preventive measures, you can significantly reduce the risk of spreading infections to yourself and others. Responsible behavior and adherence to public health guidelines play a vital role in protecting community health and preventing the transmission of infections.

Chapter 7

Alternative Treatments and Complementary Therapies

7.1 Other Antibiotics and Their Uses

There are various types of antibiotics, each with its unique spectrum of activity and specific uses. Here are some commonly used antibiotics and their respective uses:

1. Penicillins:
   - Amoxicillin: Used to treat a wide range of bacterial infections, such as respiratory tract infections, urinary tract infections, and skin infections.
   - Penicillin G: Primarily used to treat certain specific bacterial infections, such as strep throat and syphilis.
2. Cephalosporins:
   - Cephalexin: Effective against a variety of bacterial infections, including skin and soft tissue infections, urinary tract infections, and respiratory infections.
   - Ceftriaxone: Often used for severe infections or when broader coverage is needed, such as bacterial

meningitis or complicated intra-abdominal infections.

3. Macrolides:
   - Azithromycin: Used for respiratory tract infections, such as bronchitis and pneumonia, as well as certain sexually transmitted infections.
   - Clarithromycin: Used for respiratory infections, sinusitis, and certain skin infections.

4. Fluoroquinolones:
   - Ciprofloxacin: Effective against a broad range of bacterial infections, including urinary tract infections, respiratory infections, and certain gastrointestinal infections.
   - Levofloxacin: Used for respiratory infections, urinary tract infections, and skin infections.

5. Tetracyclines:
   - Doxycycline: Effective against a variety of bacterial infections, including respiratory infections, acne, and sexually transmitted infections.

6. Sulfonamides:
   - Trimethoprim-Sulfamethoxazole (Co-trimoxazole): Used for urinary

tract infections, certain respiratory infections, and some skin infections.

7. Aminoglycosides:
   - Gentamicin: Often used in combination with other antibiotics for serious infections, such as bloodstream infections and certain types of pneumonia.
8. Carbapenems:
   - Meropenem: Reserved for severe infections caused by multidrug-resistant bacteria.
9. Clindamycin:
   - Used for skin infections, respiratory infections, and dental infections.

It's essential to note that the choice of antibiotic depends on the type of infection, the bacteria involved, and the individual's health condition. The use of antibiotics should be guided by healthcare professionals, who consider factors like the patient's medical history, drug allergies, and local antibiotic resistance patterns to determine the most appropriate treatment.

7.2 Natural Remedies for Infections

Natural remedies can complement traditional medical treatments for infections and support the body's immune response. While natural remedies are not a substitute for antibiotics or other prescribed medications in severe infections, they may help with mild symptoms or in preventing infections. Here are some natural remedies that have been traditionally used:

1. Honey: Honey has antibacterial properties and can help soothe sore throats and coughs. It is commonly used to alleviate symptoms of respiratory infections.
2. Garlic: Garlic contains compounds with antimicrobial properties. It may help fight infections and support the immune system. Raw garlic is more potent, but supplements and aged garlic extract are also available.
3. Echinacea: Echinacea is a herb believed to boost the immune system and potentially reduce the severity and duration of upper respiratory infections. It is available in various forms, including teas, capsules, and extracts.
4. Elderberry: Elderberry has been used for centuries to treat colds and flu. It is believed to have antiviral properties that may help reduce symptoms and shorten the duration of viral infections.
5. Probiotics: Probiotics are beneficial bacteria that support a healthy gut microbiome. They may help strengthen the immune system

and reduce the risk of certain infections, particularly gastrointestinal infections.

6. Vitamin C: Vitamin C is an antioxidant that supports the immune system and helps the body fight infections. Citrus fruits, strawberries, kiwi, and supplements are good sources of vitamin C.

7. Zinc: Zinc is essential for immune function and may help reduce the severity and duration of colds and respiratory infections. Zinc can be found in foods like oysters, beef, and pumpkin seeds, or as a supplement.

8. Ginger: Ginger has anti-inflammatory and antimicrobial properties, making it useful for relieving symptoms of respiratory infections and upset stomachs.

9. Turmeric: Turmeric contains curcumin, which has antioxidant and anti-inflammatory properties. It may support the immune system and overall health.

10. Tea Tree Oil: Tea tree oil has natural antimicrobial properties and can be used topically for skin infections and acne.

It's essential to consult with a healthcare professional before using natural remedies, especially if you have underlying health conditions or are taking medications. Some natural remedies may interact with certain medications or have adverse effects in some individuals.

Natural remedies should not replace prescribed medications for severe infections or conditions. If you suspect you have a severe infection or are experiencing worsening symptoms, seek immediate medical attention. A healthcare provider can offer guidance on the appropriate use of natural remedies alongside conventional medical treatments.

7.3 Integrative Approaches to Healing

Integrative approaches to healing combine conventional medical treatments with complementary and alternative therapies to support overall health and well-being. These approaches aim to address the physical, emotional, mental, and spiritual aspects of health. Integrative medicine recognizes that each individual is unique and that healing requires a holistic and patient-centered approach. Some common integrative approaches to healing include:

1. Mind-Body Practices: Mind-body techniques, such as meditation, mindfulness, yoga, and tai chi, can help reduce stress, improve relaxation, and promote overall well-being. These practices are often used to complement conventional medical treatments for various conditions.

2. Nutrition and Dietary Supplements: A focus on a balanced diet, rich in nutrients, can support the body's immune system and overall health. Dietary supplements, such as vitamins, minerals, and herbal remedies, may be used to fill nutritional gaps or support specific health needs.

3. Acupuncture: Acupuncture is a traditional Chinese medicine practice that involves inserting thin needles into specific points on the body to stimulate energy flow and promote healing. It is often used to manage pain and treat various health conditions.

4. Herbal Medicine: Herbal remedies from traditional systems of medicine, such as Ayurveda, Traditional Chinese Medicine (TCM), and Native American medicine, are used to support healing and manage various health issues.

5. Chiropractic Care: Chiropractic adjustments focus on the alignment of the spine and nervous system to improve overall health and relieve pain.

6. Massage Therapy: Massage therapy can help relax muscles, reduce stress, and alleviate pain. It is often used as a complementary therapy for various medical conditions.

7. Energy Healing: Modalities like Reiki and Healing Touch work on the premise of

balancing energy flow in the body to promote healing and overall well-being.

8. Art and Music Therapy: These creative therapies can help express emotions, reduce stress, and promote mental and emotional healing.

9. Physical Therapy: Physical therapy uses exercise, manual techniques, and other interventions to rehabilitate and improve physical function after injuries or illnesses.

10. Lifestyle Modifications: Integrative medicine emphasizes the importance of healthy lifestyle habits, including regular exercise, adequate sleep, and stress management, to support overall health.

Integrative approaches to healing involve collaboration between healthcare providers and patients to develop personalized treatment plans. It is essential to communicate openly with healthcare providers about all treatments, including complementary and alternative therapies, to ensure safe and effective care.

Integrative medicine does not dismiss the value of conventional medical treatments; rather, it seeks to complement and enhance them with evidence-based complementary therapies. If you are interested in exploring integrative approaches to healing, consult with healthcare professionals experienced in integrative medicine who can provide guidance and create a comprehensive and individualized treatment plan.

Made in the USA
Monee, IL
07 February 2024

53114888R00039